Survival Medicine:
Top 15 Plants And Herbs That Will Save Your Life

Table of content

Introduction

If you step outside and open your eyes you will almost certainly see flowers and plants in abundance. Even if you live in the city you are likely to see window boxes and even a park or two on the way to and from work. All the plant life you seem is often taken for granted; many of us appreciate the beauty of it and may even marvel at how it reappears every year. However, what you may not appreciate is that some of these plants have the ability to literally save your life. This can be especially relevant if you are not near or cannot get to conventional medicine.

You may wonder, in the modern world, how it is possible for anyone to become isolated or cut off from conventional medicine. However, it is much easier than you think! Explorers and adventurers regularly go off the beaten tracks and search in places where very few people have been, but you would expect them to understand the risks of not being close to food supplied and medicine. However, anyone can find themselves stranded after a plane crash, shipwreck or even a long drive across the country. What begins as a small problem can quickly become a desperate survival issue. For instance, you are driving across a remote area of woodland, between two towns, unfortunately you car breaks down, as you wait safely beside the road for assistance you feel an urgent need to urinate so move deeper into the trees. A fog quickly comes down and you become disorientated. You start walking and when the fog clears you realize that you are completely lost. There is a good chance that a search party will be sent looking for you, but they may take several days to find you depending on where you have walked towards. Whilst you wait to be rescued you will need to survive.

One way in which you can increase your chances of survival is to know which herbs and plants can be eaten, which can be used as medicine and which should be avoided at all costs. Knowing which herbs and plants can assist you will give you an edge when it comes to surviving, whether stuck in the wilderness or after the collapse of humanity! In fact, some of the herbs listed in this book can actually be taken on a regular basis to help reduce the risk of a variety of diseases. You do not need to wait until you are stranded to start taking these. The need to survive can be applied to your everyday life as herbs which can prevent you from contracting life threatening diseases are, effectively, helping you to survive!

The most important fact to take away from this book is that now is the time to learn about which herbs are good for you and can help you survive. It is no use finding yourself in that situation and wishing you had educated yourself regarding the potential of the herbs and plants around you.

Chapter 1 – Edible Plants

The list of edible plants is huge, after all the fruit and vegetables you see in your local supermarket are all grown and can be found in the wild. The majority of these products should be familiar to you already and, if you find yourself in a survival situation, you will be happy to eat these plants which you are already familiar with. If you do need to eat plants in the wild, it is important to wash them if at all possible. This will help to remove small bacteria and any small insects which could make you ill. If you are unable to find any water then you may be able to improvise, or, you may be hungry enough that the risk is worth taking.

It is important to note that this book will provide you with fifteen herbs and plants which can help save your life. There are many more which can be used to help you; your choice in the wild will be limited by the types of plant which grows in the area you are stranded in. The better your knowledge of plant life the more likely it is that you will be able to source some food to live on.

Acorns

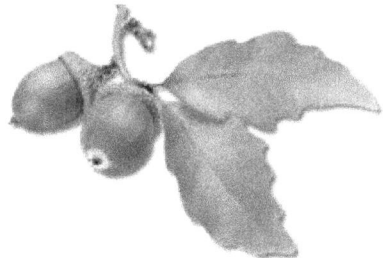

This is not something that you might usually consider eating, but they are an excellent source of protein and fat; both of which are essential to your survival. If there are oak trees in the vicinity you may find that you have a plentiful supply of acorns and this can make a huge difference to your ability to survive. Even when you are not starving it is important to eat what you can. If you do not your body will start to weaken and you will be less able to deal with simple survival tasks.

The nuts have a bitter taste and it is advisable not to consume too many of them at one time. It is also best to boil them as this will improve their flavor and make them easier to digest. The reason they taste so bitter is that they are full of tannic acid. This is not harmful but is bitter and in large quantities can give you an uncomfortable stomach.

The best method of eating acorns in the wild is to place as many as possible on a flat service as smash them with a rock. This will break their shells and you can get to the insides of them. This is the part you want to eat. You have the time it is best to soak them in warm water for a couple of hours. They are then edible; if you find they are still to bitter simply soak them for a little longer.

Dandelions

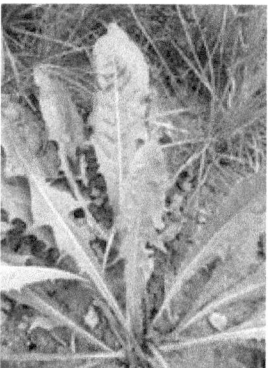

This grows almost everywhere on the planet; it is incredibly easy to recognize and surprisingly good for you. In fact, a dandelion leaf is much better for you than a standard lettuce leaf! It is known to be a plentiful supply of vitamin C, protein, fat, calcium, vitamin B, iron and even phosphorous. In fact, the humble dandelion has twelve times the amount of vitamin A that you will find in a regular lettuce leaf!

The best leaves are those which are young; although these are the smaller leaves. It is possible to eat this plant at any time of the year, although it is at its very best in the spring. It is possible to eat the leaves and even the roots if you are in a survival situation. If you are growing them at home in an attempt to add them to your diet you may wish to cut the flower heads off as early as possible; this will help the nutrition to go to the leaves and they will grow bigger. You should also protect them from the frost!

However, in the wild you can simply pull the leaves and root out of the ground and eat. It is best to wash them first; before you start looking for food you should have already found water as your body will struggle to survive for longer than a few days without water.

You can practice eating dandelion leaves at home, simply add them to a salad with your usual mixture and enjoy! It may seem like you are eating grass but this plant has a good range of nutrition which can help you stay alive.

Elderberries

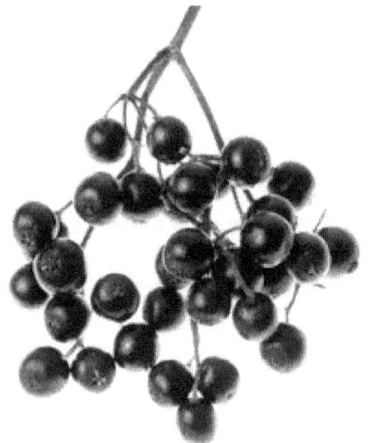

The elderberry is often overlooked when considering the variety of berries available. Traditional and better known berries, such as the blackberry or raspberry are instantly recognizable and look and taste good. In contrast the elderberry is small, very dark in color and has the potential to kill you if you do not prepare them properly!

A single shrub in the wild can easily reach ten feet and will have hundreds of berries on. It should be recognizable by its long stems with seven leaves at the end of each one. Each leaf is long and round with serrated edges. The berries are ready to be consumed in September time, obviously meaning that this survival food is seasonal. The berries are produced from the clusters of flowers which are shaped like small umbrellas. The flowers should be present in the spring and this is the best time for you to identify the plant. You will then know what you are looking for, if it becomes a necessity to eat the berries.

The berry is actually sweet and enjoyable, you can simply pick them and eat them, although be sure to check for bugs. Ideally wash them before you eat them. You should also be aware that they will turn your skin pink; although this is not a major concern when trying to survive.

Burdock

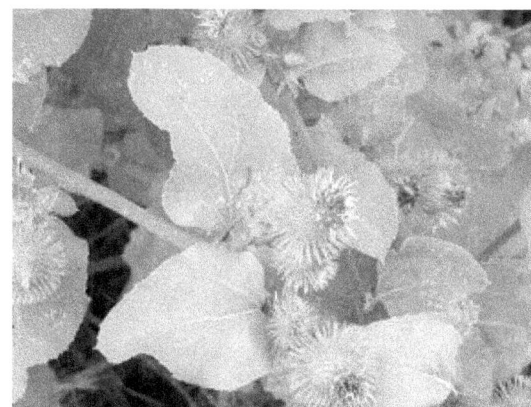

You have probably heard the words dandelion and burdock mentioned together and they are certainly both edible. The Burdock plant is medium size, towering over many weeds and comparable in size to the thistle. It also has a purple flower which bears some similarities to the standard, well known and recognized thistle. However, it does not have the large prickles of a thistle plant although the stem itself can feel prickly.

The leaves of the plant tend to be large with dips along each edge; creating an almost wrinkled effect. Originally the plant was only found in the Eastern hemisphere but it is now a common sight in many parts of the western parts of the world. It is possible to eat the leaves and the stalks, although it is necessary to peel the stalk first. You can safely eat the plant raw, however, it will taste better if it is boiled twice; this will remove the bitter taste of the leaves. It is also possible to eat the root; again you should peel it and then boil it.

Boiling may destroy some of the nutrients in any plant or herb, but, it will also help to ensure any bugs and bacteria are destroyed before you consume it. This is important as eating these plants is supposed to help you survive, not make you ill!

Cattail

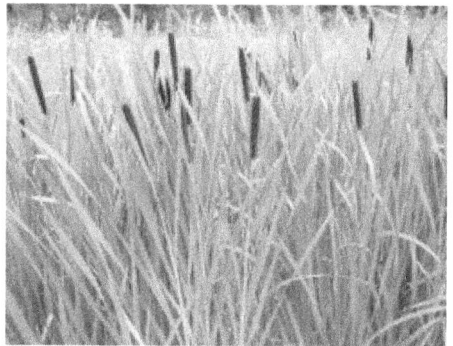

The Latin name of this plant is Typha, although it is also known as bulrush, reedmace and even punks; but you may simply refer to it as grass. It is a common sight in America, England and many other western countries. In general you will find it along the edge of the marshland; but only freshwater wetlands! This means you will need to take additional care if you are harvesting it to eat. It is possible the ground could sink under your feet, trapping you. Depending upon your location it is also possible there will be other predators in the fresh water.

If you remove the entire plant you will be able to wash the roots and eat this; it is important to wash it as you can eat this part raw. If you break the plant near the top of the root you will find that this part is the tastiest. It should appear almost completely white.

It is also possible to boil the stem and the leaves; they can then be consumed and are actually surprisingly tasty! If you are lucky enough to come across the plant in the beginning of the summer you will find that many of them have a flower which looks a little like a small corn dog. This part is also edible and can be eaten raw.

Eat it in the same way as you would a corn on the cob; in fact, it even tastes a little like corn on the cob!

Chapter 2 – 5 Herbs Which Can Help You Stay Alive

The first chapter has dealt with plants that you can find in the wild; these are a natural food source and a valuable means of surviving whilst waiting for rescue or making your own way to civilization. However, plants are only one option; the following herbs can also help you to survive. Some of these may also help your food to be more palatable, but they will all help you to survive.

Plantain

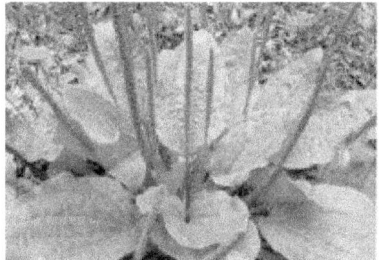

This picture shows the broad leaf variety of plantain; it is something that you are likely to have seen before as it grows almost anywhere. There is a narrow leaf version of this plant which can also be used as is just as easy to find.

The leaves can be simply picked, washed and eaten; if you combine with the nuts and berries you have already selected you will have a healthy salad which is full of valuable nutrients. Alternatively you can soak the leaf in hot water to create a tasty tea; or even use the tea to wash your skin; it is a very effective body scrub!

The herb is also known to assist with treating flu or flu like symptoms, ideally soak one whole plant in a pan of boiling water for ten minutes before drinking.

Finally, plantain is also useful for treating wounds and even burns. Smash the plant into pulp and apply this to the injured area. It will be both soothing and cleaning.

Chickweed

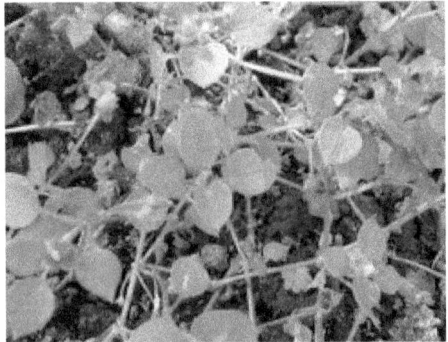

This edible plant can be called an herb or a weed. In fact it is often referred to as a weed because of the speed at which it can spread. You will probably find some of this in your garden and there will certainly be a significant quantity in the wild near you. It generally grows during the spring months although it can often be found throughout the summer months. In essence it is similar to a mild lettuce. The taste is simple, mild and yet fresh, but most importantly when surviving in the wild, it is easy to find, pick and eat. It is also full of nutrition and will help you to stay focused on the task in hand.

Again, this can be treated in much the same way as any salad leaf; you can eat it raw or mix it with any other ingredients you have to create a tasty survival dish. If you are brave enough, adding a few small grubs will really increase your protein levels and help your body to function despite the circumstances you find yourself in.

You will generally find large clumps of chickweed growing together; it will be between two inches and ten inches tall and will appear like a carpet underfoot. Chickweed is a good source of vitamin A, C and all the B's; it also provides a good mixture of metals and calcium. It has been used in the past to treat stomach upsets, circulation issues and even inflammations and blood disorders. It can also be crushed up and applied to wounds to act as an antibacterial potion.

It is worth noting that chickweed bears a startling resemblance to scarlet pimpernel. Whilst chickweed is a good source of nutrition, scarlet pimpernel is poisonous. The decisive test to confirm you have chickweed is to hold it up to the light. There will be a fine line of hairs visible on one side of the stem. It may alternate sides as it moves up or down the plant. If it does not have these hairs, do not eat it!

Wood Sorrel

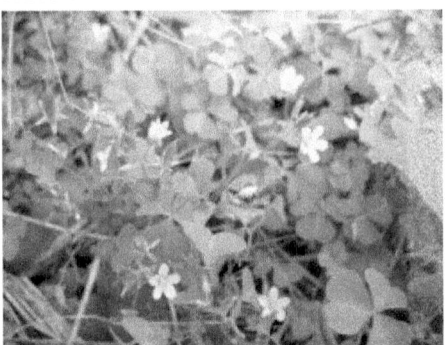

This herb is another one which is both edible and offers assistance with health issues. The plant is generally very easy to identify and, once you have sampled them the taste is not something you will forget quickly.

It looks a little like clover with the leaves appearing on opposing sides of the stem. Each set of leaves appears to be three heart shapes. Although the plant has two variants; the yellow wood sorrel and the creeping red wood sorrel, both varieties have the same yellow flowers. Each flower is like a small five pointed star, approximately half a cm wide. The stem of the plant will also be covered in microscopic hairs; you will only see these if you look exceptionally closely.

The plant can be eaten whole and raw; it tastes sour but not in an unpleasant way. In many ways you might believe you are actually eating a lemon!

It also has several medicinal qualities; it can be ground and put onto a wound to help prevent infection and to cool a burn. It can also help to regulate the kidneys and for this reason it should be avoided by anyone suffering from kidney issues. Of course, if you are trying to survive in the wild you may not be able to be too picky; in which case it should only be consumed in small amounts. It can also help to constrict your blood vessels which can be useful if you need to stop a bleed.

Another side effect of consuming too much sorrel is that it will aid the procession of food through your body and is likely to give you diarrhea; not something you want when trying to survive in the wild!

Henbit

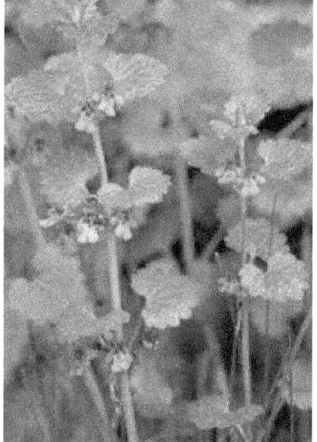

This herb is often overlooked although it can be a valuable aid when faced with a survival situation. It is very similar to purple dead nettle; however, you do not need to worry if you pick the wrong one. Dead nettle can be eaten and handled in the same as henbit, in fact, it has a similar flavor.

This herb is actually part of the mint family. It is usually recognized from the tiny flowers which are a light purple, almost pink color. The flower will appear from the middle of March until early June. The leaves are small and scallop shaped and can be eaten at any time of the year.

Despite being part of the mint family the flavor you will get from this herb is more like the taste of a lettuce leaf than mint. It is high in iron and a number of vitamins. It is also full of fiber which can help you to feel fuller for longer; something that may help you when trying to survive.

You can eat the stem and the leaves raw, or you can add them to other dishes to add a little extra flavor. It can also be soaked in hot water to make a delicious cup of tea.

Sow Thistle

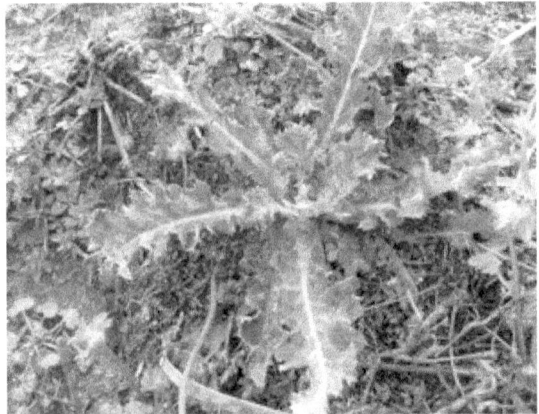

The sow thistle is usually classed as a weed, although it is, in fact, an herb. It does not look particularly appetizing as it is covered in spiny leaves. In fact, this plant has very similar properties to the dandelion, even the flower looks similar! However, you will notice the difference if you grab it quickly; the small sharp leaves will remind you of their presence.

In fact, the leaves are quite tasty. They can be eaten in the same way as a dandelion but it is essential to remove the spikes first. You can do this by pulling each one out or simply running your pocket knife around the edge of the leaf. This will cut the ends of the leaves off and leave it safe for you to eat. Even the stalks can be peeled and eaten; you will find they have a consistency similar to celery, although the taste is noticeable different.

The plant has also been acknowledged as having healing properties. It has been brewed as a tea to help remove obstructions in the urinary tract and allow comfortable urination.

As with the dandelion leaf there are a mixture of important vitamins and metals which can be obtained by eating this plant.

Chapter 3 – 5 Medicinal Herbs

Being isolated in a wilderness scenario is daunting at the best of times, but the situation can often be made much worse if you are feeling ill or have injured yourself. This can often be the case if the incident has happened suddenly and is the result of an accident. However, an injury can serious affect your ability to forage properly and may even make you a more attractive target for predators. Unfortunately once you are isolated in the wild you are much more at risk from a variety of large animals.

As well as impeding any survival attempt or your ability to travel, an injury can result in infection and consequent illness. Without antibiotics you can even find yourself succumbing to blood poisoning or other infections which are usually easily treated.

This is not a new skill; medicinal herbs have been used for generations; long before modern drugs and chemicals were created. They can be used to great effect. To ensure you are able to deal with any situation it is essential to learn which herbs can be used to treat these conditions:

Aloe Leaf

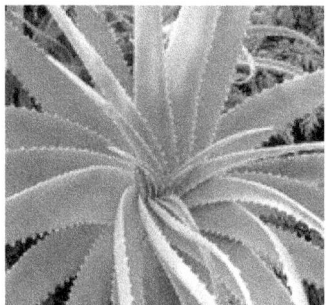

The Aloe leaf is where one of the most familiar of natural remedies comes from; aloe vera. It has been used in skin creams, sunburn lotions and even added to moisturizers and has a myriad of uses. The plant can also be found in the wild and can be a valuable benefit if you have any one of a number of injuries.

To get the valuable aloe vera lotion you will need to carefully pull a leaf of the plant and then trim all the prickles off from the leaf. You will then be able to split the leaf in half without injuring yourself further!

The exposed sap can be rubbed onto a wound, burn or even unknown skin disorders. The gel will rapidly cool and sooth the affected area allowing the body to start the healing process. It will also act as a barrier to germs and other bacteria; helping to ensure your cut does not result in an infection. It has been proven to speed up the healing process and may make the difference between you being able to forage for food or not.

Comfrey Leaf

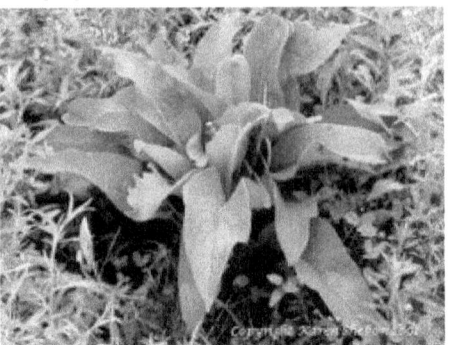

The comfrey leaf has been used in Chinese medicine for thousands of years. However, more recent research suggests that continued use of this herb internally may be toxic as it can cause damage to your liver. As you will be using this in a survival situation this is not generally an issue. It is also possible to simply use it to help with healing externally.

The leaf has been shown to help stop bleeding and can even encourage your tissues to regenerate; speeding the time it takes for your body to repair itself. The leaves can be ground into a paste and then applied to the skin, either directly to a cut or over the site of a fractured bone. It will soak into the body and help your injured bone heal. It is even effective if you apply it to muscles and tendons which you have pulled or strained.

It is important to note that the comfrey leaf is incredibly fast acting. Any cut will be sealed in moments; effectively trapping any dirt or bacteria in the wound. You must be certain the wound is clean before you seal it with this herb. If it is still bleeding then this is a good sign that the wound is clean as any debris or bacteria are likely to be carried out with the blood.

St. John's Wort

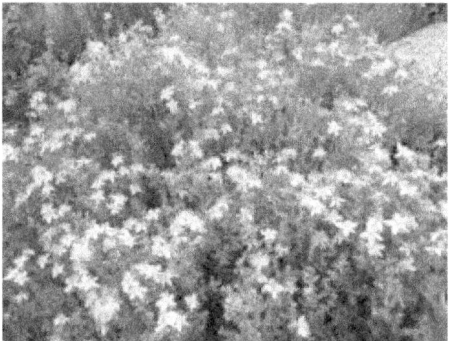

This is another natural herb which is present in a wide variety of over the counter products. It can even be bought in liquid form. The plant grows almost anywhere, it will quickly spread and cover any spare land with its green stems and bright yellow flowers. If left, they will grow to waist height relatively quickly.

The best part to use when in the wild is the flower bud, not the flower itself. This can be crushed and it will produce a liquid which is red, bordering on purple. This liquid can then be applied directly to an injured area to provide plain relief. In fact St. John's Wort is a very effective pain reliever as it targets the nerves directly. It will actively encourage your nerves to start healing and reduce the pain in the process.

It is possible to harvest the buds in the summer and mix them with olive oil which can then be drunk to assist with pain killing. However, this is unlikely to be an option in the wild.

An additional benefit of St. John's Wort is that it is naturally an anti-depressant. This may seem trivial but anything which can help; to keep your spirits up in a survival situation will be of benefit!

Yarrow

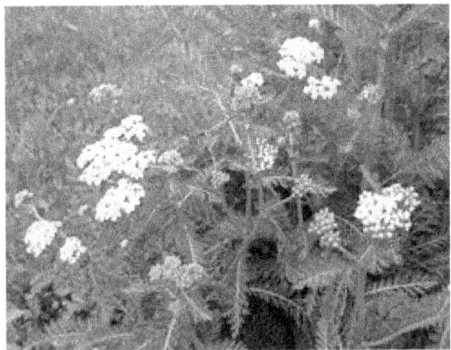

This plant can be found in many parts of the world and is easy to distinguish thanks to its fern like leaves and clusters of white flowers. It is an exceptionally good way of stopping bleeding; this will allow you to treat your wound and start recovering. Blood will also attract predators so it is advisable to move on as soon as you have stopped the bleeding.

You can make a paste from the flowers by crushing them; between two rocks or even between your fingers. The paste can be applied directly to a wound to stop the bleeding.

It has also been used to make tea by brewing in hot water for a minimum of five minutes. The tea is effective at treating colds, fevers and a range of digestive problems. It should not be taken over an extended period of time as it can be toxic.

Jewelweed

This plant has tall slim stems with a flower hanging off the top; in many ways it has the appearance of a jewel hanging on a necklace; in fact, this I how the plant got its name. It has been used for many years to treat outbreaks of poison ivy, although it is effective against almost any kind of plant based rash. To use this in the wild you will need to squeeze or crush the stem and even the leaves; this will produce a clear liquid which can be used to gently rub on the affected area. The soothing effects of this plant will be felt almost immediately; allowing you to focus on more important survival tasks.

The extract from this plant is also effective when used to treat bruises, burns and even cuts. It has even been effective at taking away the soreness of an insect bite; something which could prove very valuable when in the wilderness.

It is also interesting to note that the jewelweed is often found growing near poison ivy; as though nature has provided the cure ready for you!

Conclusion

This book has merely touched on the number of herbs and plants which are available in the wild and can be used to aid survival. There are many more. However, it is important to study these plants now and be certain you know what you are looking at. There are many plants which can benefit your health but which look very similar to ones which will make you ill, or even kill you. By studying these plants now you will have no issue when needing them to survive.

It is quite possible that you will have heard it said that humans can go for weeks and sometimes even months without food, providing they have water. If you have no water you will be unlikely to survive longer than three or five days. This means that if you are in a survival situation water and shelter are the most important things.

But, once you have found these, it remains an important goal to source food. If you do not your body will go into fasting mode, you will immediately notice the affect of this and will have less energy and less motivation. Eating even small amounts of food per day will keep your body from moving into this mode and provide important nutritional benefit. Perhaps even more importantly will be the psychological and emotional effect. Being able to source food and locate plants to help treat any injuries will provide you with a mental lift. You will know it is possible to survive in the wilderness; instead of wondering if you will ever be rescued or if you will die alone in the wilderness, you will be considering the best plan to take you back to civilization. Water and shelter are essential physical needs; food is the essential emotional lift which will get you home.

Of course, there are plenty of plants which will harm you and the golden rule is if you are not sure to leave them alone. However, if your hunger increases and you have not had any success finding the plants and herbs you do know about then it is important to avoid any plant which displays the following symptoms:

- Colored sap; in general a plant with clear sap will be safe to eat; although wherever possible you should wash or boil it first.

- Thorny or spiky plants are usually dangerous; this is nature's way of warning people and animals to stay away from them. This is not always true but if you are unfamiliar with a specific plant it is best to err on the side of caution.

- Taste; ideally you should try as many of the plants you are likely to encounter and may need to rely on before you go on a trip. If you are sampling plants it is best to ensure your palate is clear first. This will ensure you obtain the full flavor. The benefit of doing this now is that if you are stuck in the wild you will be able to taste a very small part of a plant and know whether it tastes like it should. If it does not then you should not eat it.

- Mushrooms are exceptionally hard to calculate whether they are okay to eat or not. There are many different species and some of the nicest ones look very similar to some of the deadliest ones! If you do find mushrooms and you believe they are edible it is best to try a small piece and then wait, ideally for twenty four hours, before you have any more.

Knowing which plants and herbs have medicinal properties can be as important as food, any injury you receive in the wild will be far worse than one in a civilized area simply because you will not have access to medical care. There are plants which can stop the bleeding, provide pain relief and even act as an antiseptic; providing you know what you are looking for.

There is a marked increase in the ability to live off the land and an abundance of information. Once you have mastered the basics illustrated in this book you will be able to advance your learning; it is a fascinating subject!

FREE Bonus Reminder

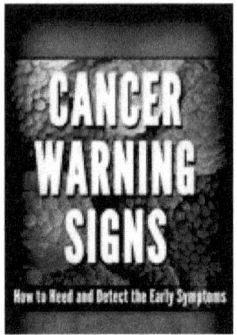

If you have not grabbed it yet, please go ahead and download your special bonus report *"DIY Projects. 13 Useful & Easy To Make DIY Projects To Save Money & Improve Your Home!"*

Simply Click the Button Below

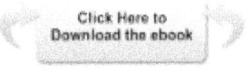

OR Go to This Page

http://healthylivingpeople.com/free/

BONUS #2: More Free & Discounted Books

Do you want to receive more Free & Discounted Books?

We have a mailing list where we send out our new Books when they go free or with a discount on Kindle. Click on the link below to sign up for Free & Discount Book Promotions.

=> Sign Up for Free & Discount Book Promotions <=

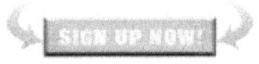

OR Go to this URL

http://zbit.ly/1WBb1Ek